WHAT EVERY ABOUT SEEDING

A PERSONAL CHOICE: SEEDING VERSUS SURGERY

When I was diagnosed with a Stage B2 prostate cancer in 1990, radioactive seed implantation (brachytherapy) was still considered investigational, and there was very little information available to patients about their treatment options. Radical surgery (prostatectomy) was considered the "gold standard" treatment for early stage cases like mine. The PSA blood test had only been in use for a few years; in fact, I didn't even have a PSA reading prior to being treated.

A lot has changed since 1990. PSA testing has transformed the entire field of prostate cancer therapy by enabling doctors to determine the cure rates for every type of treatment at an earlier time. More rigorous standards must now be met before a patient is considered cured. Indeed, the medical community has been shocked to discover that cure rates following all forms of treatment are not as high as previously believed. Early stage cancers, which were thought to be curable in more than 90 percent of patients, have turned out to be curable in only about 50-70 percent of cases. This is true of both radical prostatectomy and conventional external beam radiation therapy.

In contrast, the cure rates with seed implantation appear to be as high as 90 percent at five years and longer, according to recent reports. Moreover, the risk of permanent side effects with seeding is low. Improved results are also being reported with a new hi-tech form of external radiation, known as "conformal radiation." In some cases, conformal radiation is being combined with seed implantation for high risk patients.

I have a special interest in seeding because this was the type of therapy that I chose over surgery. At the time I made my choice, the promising results of the 5-year studies (1994) on seed implants had not yet been reported; but I was determined to avoid, if possible, the risks of surgical side effects such as sexual impotence and incontinence. When first diagnosed, I was 44 years old, a family man with children still in diapers. As I faced the crisis over a period of months and explored my options, preserving my quality of life was a personal priority as important to me as curing my cancer.

Seeding made the most sense to me once I learned about the procedure, and how it has been refined during recent years. In retrospect, I have no regrets whatsoever about the choice I made.

I had 63 seeds of Palladium-103 implanted without experiencing any of the complications or permanent side effects often associated with surgery. I have been cancer-free for almost six years, and my most recent PSA reading was .019 ng/ml. With each passing year, I have become more convinced that I am cured, that I made the right choice. Because of my positive experience and the results now being reported with seeding, I wrote a book on the subject (***Prostate Cancer: A Survivor's Guide***), and I continue to encourage men to seriously consider this option before embarking on any course of action.

Seeding is not appropriate for every patient, and I have written this booklet to answer the most common questions about the procedure, and to help you decide if seeding is right for you. Before deciding on any treatment, you should fully investigate the likelihood of cure, and the risk of side effects that may alter your quality of life. These are the most important considerations in deciding on treatment. Given your age, your overall health, and the stage of the cancer, you will want to find a balance between effectiveness and side effects -- a balance with which you are comfortable, that you can live with both before and after treatment. Knowing what to expect each step of the way is one of the keys to fighting this disease.

You should also be aware that much of the information available on prostate cancer has been written with a definite pro-surgical bias. It is not surprising that surgeons recommend surgery, especially in light of the old saw that the best way to fight cancer is simply to cut it out. However, with prostate cancer, as with breast cancer, the traditional wisdom of radical surgery is more and more in doubt. Fortunately, you do have a choice, with the emergence of promising, state-of-the-art treatment options, such as seed implantation.

As you read this booklet and continue your research, keep in mind that you should carefully examine the pros and cons of **all** options before embarking on any course of treatment.

WHAT IS SEEDING?

Also called "interstitial implantation therapy" (or brachytherapy), this treatment involves the insertion of radioactive seeds into the prostate gland. The radioactive seeds can either be inserted temporarily, or can remain permanently in place within the prostate. These permanent seeds pose no health threat to the patient, and decay within 6 months to a year, becoming inert and inactive.

Since being developed in the 1970's and 1980's as an investigational technique, seed implantation has become widely available in the United States. A number of technical refinements in the procedure have led to improved results and increasing popularity. Seeding is now available at several hundred medical centers throughout the country.

In the old days, seed implants required major abdominal surgery. Seeds of radioactive isotopes were manually implanted into the prostate using needles, but the procedure achieved poor results because of a lack of precision in placing the seeds. Poor placement led to "cold" spots within the prostate gland that did not receive a sufficient dose of radiation to destroy the cancer. In more recent years, a non-invasive technique has been devised for implanting the seeds in the prostate without open surgery (known as "transperineal implantation"). Seeds are dispensed using hollow needles which are inserted through the perineum, the area between the scrotum and the anus. A template or grid is used to precisely guide the placement of the needles.

The technique has been further refined with the use of realtime imaging, often utilizing transrectal ultrasound, although sometimes using CT scanning or fluoroscopy, for dynamic visualization. With these technological improvements, a more precise, three-dimensional image of the prostate can be generated, and the seeds can be more accurately placed, where they will do the most good. The strategy has been to target and destroy the cancer with minimal exposure to surrounding tissue and organs. The computerized guidance system helps determine where the seeds should go, how deeply they should be inserted, and how strong their radiation should be.

Brachytherapy with ultrasound or fluoroscopic guidance has a number of advantages over the more conventional external beam radiation therapy. Because radiation can damage healthy tissue as well as cancerous tissue, the standard dose of radiation used externally on the prostate is approximately 7000 rads (or 70 Gray), calculated to be the highest dose which is safe and well tolerated by the patient. Seed implants deliver radiation only to the prostate itself and not to surrounding organs. As a consequence, higher doses of radiation (up to 16,000 rads, or 160 Gray) can be administered to the area of the prostate using internally implanted seeds. While the electronic grid ensures an accurate and comprehensive distribution of seeds, ultrasound and fluoroscopy are used to check and double-check the position of the seeds.

Seeding with guidance thus offers a state-of-the-art, cost effective means of treating early stage prostate cancer. The price for the procedure is about half that of radical prostatectomy, and the operation can be performed in less than an hour on an out-patient basis, making it very appealing to those men wanting to avoid the added risks and hospitalization involved in major surgery. At the very least, then, seed implants provide an excellent alternative for older patients, as well as for younger patients who wish to avoid radical surgery and the likelihood of morbidity.

A number of radiation sources have been used for interstitial implantation. The most commonly used permanent implants are encapsulated isotopes of either Iodine-125 or Palladium-103. While somewhat more expensive, Palladium-103 has a significantly shorter half-life (the period of time until its output of radiation is halved) and a greater initial radiation dose than Iodine-125. Thus, in theory, palladium may be more effective against rapidly growing, more aggressive cancers (those with higher Gleason scores). Because the radiation is active for a shorter period with palladium, temporary side effects (such as urinary distress) may also be shorter in duration.

Temporary implants utilize pellets of another isotope, Iridium-192, used in combination with a course of low or medium dose external radiation. While the temporary procedure may eventually prove to be as effective as permanent implants, it is not used as commonly because it requires a hospital stay of several days and is more expensive. There is little published data on temporary implants, but early findings appear to indicate a somewhat higher rate of complications because of the extremely penetrating, high dose of radiation delivered with this isotope.

ARE YOU A CANDIDATE FOR SEEDING?

If you are a candidate for surgery, you are probably also a candidate for seed implantation, as both treatments are most effective with early stage cancers.

In addition, many men who would not be candidates for surgery -- those patients over the age of 70, or those men with other health conditions that rule out major surgery -- may qualify as candidates for seeding, which is a much less invasive procedure than radical prostatectomy.

The most important factor in determining a patient's eligibility for seeding is how far the cancer has spread. If the cancer is localized, that is, confined to the prostate gland, then it is more likely to be curable, with either surgery or seeding. Once the cancer has spread beyond the prostate capsule, it is not curable by implantation alone, because the seed implants do not radiate enough area around the prostate to destroy any cancer that may have spread beyond the prostate capsule. In a similar way, surgery is also unlikely to cure those patients who have disease outside the prostate capsule.

Those patients with Stage A or small B tumors -- also known as Stage T1 or T2 -- are most likely to have cancer that is confined to the prostate, and therefore, curable with seed implantation alone.

Patients with larger Stage B or C (T2, T3, or T4) cancers, a high Gleason score (greater than a combined score of 6, or a single score of 4) or a high PSA (greater than 10), or an elevated PAP (enzymatic acid phosphatase) are more likely to have cancer which has extended beyond the prostate capsule (known as "extra-capsular extension"). Patients with any one of these risk factors may be treated with either high dose conformal radiation, or a combination of conformal radiation and seed implants.

Since the ideal candidates for seeding are all of those patients most likely to benefit from cure, seed implantation should be considered by all men who have cancer that appears to be confined to the prostate region, and therefore, is potentially curable. Also, it should only be considered by patients who are young enough and healthy enough to live long enough to benefit from being cured -- those patients with a life expectancy of ten years or longer. Good candidates are men from their forties to their seventies, with localized prostate cancer. Some men in their eighties who are in good health may also benefit from implantation.

Most patients are able to tolerate the seed implantation procedure, which requires only light anesthesia. Men with a history of heart disease or stroke are advised to have a thorough medical examination, including a cardiac stress test, before proceeding with the procudure. Patients who have had a portion of their prostate removed with a previous TURP (transurethral resection of the prostate) may be at increased risk for urinary incontinence after seeding. If only a small amount of tissue was removed with the TURP, then it is probably safe to proceed with implantation. Further refinements are being developed that appear to lessen the likelihood of morbidity for patients with a prior TURP. By implanting the seeds away from the urethra, the risk of urinary incontinence may be substantially reduced.

Patients with very enlarged prostates or those men who have difficulty with urination prior to treatment may have more severe urinary problems after implantation. Treatment is typically restricted to men with prostates less than 60 cubic centimeters volume. Some doctors prescribe two or three months of hormonal therapy before implantation in order to shrink the prostate.

WHAT STAGE CANCERS CAN BE TREATED WITH SEEDING?

Stage A1 (T1a): Focalized Low Grade Impalpable Tumors

The majority of A1 stage prostate cancers, perhaps as many as 85 to 90 percent -- will not become health or life threatening during the lifetime of the patient. Usually discovered following a TURP (transurethral resection of the prostate), these small, incidental tumors seldom demand any treatment other than careful observation and monitoring (watchful waiting). Men under 60, however, may be at appreciable risk of disease progression and should consider treatment at this stage.

Various studies have shown no apparent value in aggressive treatment of stage A1 prostate cancers. Radical surgery is now typically deemed inappropriate for these incidental cancers. Patients with these cancers are more likely to die "with" the cancer, not "of" the cancer. This is especially true for patients with PSA values less than 1.0. Patients with higher PSA values, especially those over 10.0, are more likely to benefit from early treatment. For these patients, seed implantation may offer a more appealing curative treatment because of the lower risk of permanent side effects.

Stage A2 (T1b): High Grade or Diffuse Impalpable Tumors

Clinically diagnosed stage A2 prostate cancers are more aggressive than stage A1, and possess a propensity to metastasize. For this reason, these cancers usually merit some form of immediate, curative treatment.

Treatments for stage A2 patients include seed implantation, as well as radical prostatectomy and external beam radiation therapy. Analysis of radical prostatectomy specimens has shown that as many as 50 percent of patients will have cancer that has extended beyond the confines of the prostate, and thus, cannot be said to be cured by the procedure, even though the cancer may not recur.

Conventional external radiation therapy has achieved results roughly equivalent to surgery. Studies suggest that many if not most men treated with external radiation will have residual cancer, but disease progression may not occur for a decade or more. These results may be improved with hi-tech "conformal" radiation. Using three-dimensional, computerized methods, a higher total radiation dose can be externally delivered to the prostate while minimizing exposure to nearby organs. These methods represent a significant technical advance in radiation therapy, and the early results appear promising.

Seed implantation has demonstrated an ability to control cancer in stage A2 patients over the 5-year period that is comparable or superior to either surgery or conventional external radiation therapy, when the results of each type of treatment are compared at similar times. Studies done at Seattle's Northwest Tumor Institute, Tampa's University Community Hospital, and

New York's Memorial Sloan Kettering Cancer Center have reported success rates 80-90 percent for early stage tumors (using clinical and PSA normalization as end criteria for assessing cure).

While these results are impressive, it should be noted that 5 to 10 years is still a limited time period for evaluating a cancer that grows as slowly as prostate cancer. Nevertheless, this is the duration of time in which all therapies, including radical surgery, are being evaluated using the latest techniques and most rigorous standards for cure. In part, this is so because monitoring with PSA following treatment has been the standard practice only for the past decade or so.

Stage T1C: Impalpable Tumurs Identified By Needle Biopsy After Elevated PSA

These are cancers that are confirmed by biopsy after the patient shows an elevated PSA reading. If the PSA value and Gleason score are low, some of these patients may be candidates for watchful waiting. Others with higher PSA values and higher Gleason scores may be good candidates for early, curative treatment, including seed implantation (see the detailed comments for stage A (T1a) above, as they apply to T1c stage as well).

Stage B1 (T2a/T2b): Focalized Palpable Tumor Involving One Lobe Or Less

Moderate or high grade B1 cancer is less likely to have extended to the lymph nodes than A2 stage cancer. This is an encouraging finding, since those with lymph node or seminal vesicle involvement have a significantly worse prognosis. Aggressive treatment may be most advantageous for patients with B1 tumors, because the chances for cure are good, and in most cases the disease will eventually become life threatening.

Men in their seventies or older may be candidates for watchful waiting, especially if overall health mitigates against more aggressive treatment. The effectiveness of surgical treatment is well established, as two-thirds or more of men treated will live 10 years without recurrence. Only 10 to 15 percent of men will die from recurrence at 15 years. External radiation therapy and implantation have demonstrated similar therapeutic results, even though long term cure has yet to be demonstrated with these treatments (see comments above for stage A2 cancers). Again, the medium term results with seeding and the reduced risk of permanent side effects make this an appealing alternative for men wishing to avoid the risks associated with radical surgery. A 5-year study by the Northwest Tumor Institute has followed 320 patients, the majority with stage B1(T2a) cancer. 87 percent of these patients were free of disease and had PSA levels less than 1.0.

Stage B2 (T2c): Palpable Tumor Involving More Than Half the Prostate

Stage B2 cancer is the most advanced stage of cancer still clinically confined to the prostate gland. Treatment for these cancers is complicated by the difficulty in clinically assessing whether the cancer has penetrated the prostate capsule, in which case it should be classified as a stage C (T3, T4) cancer. Many of these stage B2 cancers are understaged, as evidenced by the examination of prostatectomy specimens. Studies suggest that as many as 60 percent or more of patients initially diagnosed with B2 cancers will actually have stage C (cancer extending beyond the prostate capsule) or stage D1 (positive lymph nodes).

As these understaged B2 cancers are actually not localized, they are not as effectively treated with radical surgery as stage B1 cancers. The nerve-sparing surgical technique fared poorly in at least one sample group, with only 25 percent of patients having both complete removal of the tumor and preservation of potency. Even so, one study shows about half will survive 10 years with no recurrence of cancer. External radiation therapy has generated similar 5 and 10 year results. However, local failure (as indicated by PSA and/or biopsy) appears higher, and recurrence of cancer may continue beyond 10 years, suggesting that cure may be less likely.

Recent results with seed implants have proven more successful. Using PSA to measure treatment effectiveness, ultrasound or fluoroscopically guided seed implantation has compared very favorably with other forms of treatment, with reduced risk of permanent side effects. Stage B2 patients are also candidates for seeding combined with conformal radiation, with promising results now being reported.

Stage C (T3, T4): Tumor No Longer Confined to Prostate

Stage C cancers present many difficulties, since prostate cancer is considered by most physicians to be incurable once it has extended beyond the prostate gland. Radical prostatectomy has proven ineffective in treating stage C patients. At least half of those with stage C cancer have tumorous pelvic lymph nodes upon dissection and examination, and will not benefit from radical surgery. Studies are ongoing that attempt to "downstage" stage C cancers to stage B with the use of hormonal therapy, before radical prostatectomy. But examination of surgical specimens from these patients still show extension of cancer beyond the prostate capsule or at the point of surgical resection.

External beam radiation therapy has been the most accepted lone therapy in treatment of stage C cancers. Studies are also underway on the use of hormonal therapy combined with external radiation. Combining seed implantation with low dose conformal radiotherapy has achieved impressive short-term results with lower morbidity than radiation alone. Radioactive seed implantation used as the sole therapy has resulted in high recurrence rates, and does not appear to be an effective treatment for stage C patients.

Stage D1, D2 (N+, M+): Advanced Metastatic Disease

Stage D1 and D2 cancers are those that have spread to the lymph nodes and to the bones, respectively. Patients with D1 and D2 cancers are generally not appropriate for curative therapies, including seed implantation. This does not mean that there are not treatments for men with advanced stage disease. There are treatments for fighting the disease, such as hormonal therapy, orchiectomy (castration), and chemotherapy. One recent report even suggests that some D1 patients may benefit from a concurrent therapy of hormones and radiation (either conformal alone or combined with seeding).

HOW EFFECTIVE IS SEEDING AT CURING LOCALIZED CANCER?

It is worth repeating that medium term results (5 years) with seed implantation have proven to be comparable or superior to the best surgical results for Stage A and B cancers. This is especially significant since these results are based on the more sensitive PSA success rates.

Overall, about 60 to 90 percent of these early stage patients remain cancer-free depending on factors such as pre-treatment PSA values and Gleason scores. Men with higher Gleason scores and higher PSA values are somewhat less likely to be cured by seed implantation alone. Some of these high risk patients, and some patients with stage C cancers may benefit from seed implantation combined with conformal radiation therapy.

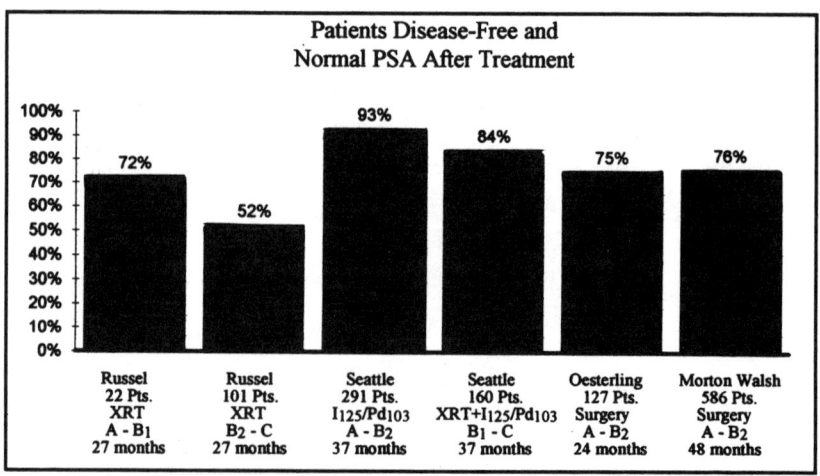

Figure 1. Comparison of prostate cancer treatments using the PSA test as an indicator of treatment effectiveness. Number of patients, form of treatment, and the stages treated are shown. Average follow-up period is shown in months. *(Courtesy J. Blasko, M.D., H. Ragde, M.D., and P. Grimm, D.O.)*

WHAT HAPPENS BEFORE THE SEEDING PROCEDURE?

To plan an implant, images of the prostate are analyzed a few days before (in my case, the day before) using ultrasound or CT scanning. The images are used to calculate the volume and position of the prostate in the body, an essential part of the preplanning stage of the procedure. The data generated is analyzed using a computer to determine the optimal dose of radiation and proper distribution of the seeds, either iodine or palladium.

The precise and specialized preparation involved in this procedure results in a treatment plan individualized to the patient. The number of seeds implanted, the number of implant needles used, and the exact configuration used in the placement of the seeds all vary according to the needs of the specific patient. This careful planning ensures that the optimal level of radiation is delivered to all areas of the patient's prostate.

Often with the aid of a physicist, the doctor will prepare the template and implant needles before the operation, based on your individualized treatment plan. To prepare for the procedure, the seeds or pellets, which look like tiny pieces of pencil lead, are inserted into the implant needles. The number of seeds per needle can vary from two to five. Each needle is numbered according to the corresponding hole in the template into which it is to be inserted. The template itself is a square Lexan plate. The holes in this plate guide the needles as they are inserted into the prostate gland, where the seeds are then deposited.

WHAT HAPPENS DURING THE SEEDING PROCEDURE?

The entire procedure can be performed in about an hour, and it is often done on an outpatient basis, meaning that the patient can come into the hospital in the morning, undergo the procedure, and be sent home a few hours later. As a matter of protocol, some physicians have their patients stay one night in the hospital. The implant procedure is non-invasive, meaning that no incisions are made. The patient is usually given the option of local or general anesthesia, as either can be used.

To begin the procedure, the patient is placed on an operating table in what is called the "lithotomy position." This is a fancy way of saying you are on your back with your legs up in stirrups. The extended position of the legs allows for placement of the seeds in the anterior of the prostate, while avoiding the pubic bones.

Once in position, patients who choose local anesthesia will be given an injection. You may also receive an injection of dexamethasone, which helps prevent acute urinary retention. The needle guide template is then positioned flush with the perineum, the area directly between the legs.

Once the anesthesia is started, a urinary catheter (a thin, flexible tube) may be inserted through the penis into the bladder, to drain urine from the bladder during and immediately after the operation. An ultrasound probe is inserted into the rectum. Both the catheter and ultrasound probe will be removed once the procedure is complete.

During the procedure, the needle positions are carefully checked and double-checked using ultrasound and/or x-rays to make sure they are in the right place. If they are improperly positioned, the needles will be removed, and the position of the guide template will then be adjusted, so the needles can be reinserted. Once the needles are properly positioned, each needle is inserted into the prostate to a depth previously determined by the computerized treatment plan. The seeds are injected through the needles as the sleeves of the needles are withdrawn, leaving the seeds implanted within the prostate. The seeds will appear as rows of tiny white dashes on an ultrasound monitor.

Once all of the seeds are in place, the procedure is complete, and the patient is usually given several hours to recover and allow the anesthesia to wear off. During that time, the catheter is removed, and an ice pack may be used to minimize swelling in the crotch area where the seeds were inserted.

Most patients do not experience any discomfort during the procedure, either with the catheter or with the needle implantation. In fact, many patients remain unaware that they have undergone the procedure even after they are in the recovery room. It is not unusual for a recovering patient to ask his doctor when he is going to begin the operation.

WHAT HAPPENS AFTER THE SEEDING PROCEDURE?

Patients are routinely monitored the day after the procedure. CT scans and X-rays are used to check the placement of the seeds. Additional medication to avoid urinary retention may be administered.

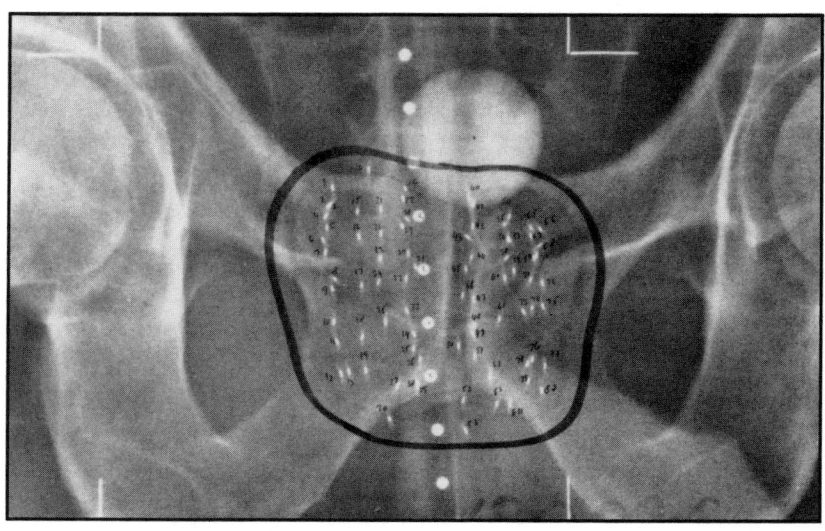

Figure 2. An x-ray of the prostate following brachytherapy. As shown in the photo, the seeds are carefully numbered and accounted for as part of the follow-up procedure. *(Courtesy of Theragenics, Inc.)*

Many patients experience some urinary burning for at least one or two days after the procedure, but most patients do not require pain medication. During the first night after the procedure, many patients experience frequent urination, perhaps as often as every hour or two, because of irritation caused by the insertion of the needles. This discomfort may be avoided by patients who stay in the hospital for care overnight. Many men will also pass some blood in their urine or ejaculation fluid for a few days after treatment.

These are temporary side effects that clear up quickly for most patients. Excessive bleeding almost never occurs. The risk of infection is minimal, but your doctor will probably prescribe antibiotics as a precaution. Patients are cautioned to avoid heavy lifting or excessive physical exertion for several days after the procedure. But otherwise, most patients can resume normal activities.

Because of the implanted radiation, whether the source is iodine or palladium, patients are advised to exercise caution with young children under the age of two, and with women who are pregnant. A young child should not be seated on a patient's lap for a prolonged period, and the same applies to a pregnant woman. Casual contact poses no health risks.

These precautions to protect children and pregnant women should be observed for a period of two to six months depending on the isotope used. The seeds will not set off the alarms of metal detectors.

Occasionally, a seed or two may become dislodged and be passed out in the urine. You may find such a seed in the bottom of the toilet or on the bathroom floor. Your doctor will instruct you on care in handling a displaced seed, and may suggest that you place a retrieved seed in a jar and return it to his office. Some doctors advise straining the urine for a short period to recover displaced seeds. As a seed might also be passed in the ejaculate fluid, patients are advised to use a condom during sex for one to several months after the procedure. Fortunately, because of the comprehensive planning of the procedure, saturating the prostate with seeds, any displaced seeds should not have to be re-implanted. For instructions on handling displaced seeds, patients are advised to call the radiation therapy department at the hospital where the procedure was performed.

WHAT ARE THE POSSIBLE SIDE EFFECTS OF SEEDING?

Seed implantation involves significantly less risk of complications compared with surgery. Side effects with seeding are usually mild and temporary. As the radioactive sources decay, some men suffer urinary problems such as urgency, frequency or difficulty in urinating. These symptoms generally dissipate by the time the seeds have lost their radioactivity. In some men, such symptoms may continue six months or longer. Some rectal irritation and bleeding may also occur over the same period. Incontinence and other serious complications are rare, except in those patients who have undergone a TURP procedure in the past.

General radiation side effects are unlikely with seed implantation because the radiation is confined to such a small part of the body. Some minimal fatigue may occur. Patients do not experience more serious radiation side effects such as hair loss, nausea, vomiting, or chronic diarrhea.

While side effects with implantation are usually temporary, it should be noted that there is some risk of more serious, permanent complications, including urinary incontinence, rectal damage, and sexual impotence. When they do occur, it is usually 6 to 24 months after treatment.

Urinary Symptoms and Complications

The urinary side effects of seeding can be severe in some men. The radiation causes inflammation of the prostate and urethra, which may lead to frequent urination, most intense at night, when patients may have to urinate every hour or two for several months or more after the procedure. Others may experience difficulty in starting their urine stream.

There is often a greater urgency to urinate, and as such, when the impulse to urinate is felt, a patient wants to relieve himself as quickly as possible. Urgency may be experienced by some men for months, when the radiation is most active. With iodine, urinary symptoms usually reach a peak at 4 to 6 weeks after treatment, then subside over the next 3 to 12 months. With palladium, symptoms may appear earlier, and they may subside more quickly because of its shorter half life.

Again, these are temporary symptoms that can vary from man to man. Permanent urinary complications are much less common. Urinary incontinence affects less than 1 percent of all patients, usually those who have had a TURP in the past. Incontinence refers to an inability to hold one's urine. Loss of bladder control ranges from mild incontinence (leaking a few drops under stress of physical exertion) to severe incontinence, in which the patient experiences a total loss of control. Even with these severe cases, which are rare, exercises, medications, or surgical intervention may be used to restore urinary control to the patient.

Rectal Symptoms and Complications

Implant radiation often causes temporary inflammation of a small area of the rectum adjacent to the prostate. Discomfort may be experienced when the patient is having a bowel movement, and this irritation may persist for several months. The patient may also have more frequent bowel movements, perhaps two or three times a day. Rectal irritability is generally not accompanied by diarrhea. The symptoms usually begin a few weeks after treatment, and may continue for 3 to 6 months.

Because seeds deliver a high dose of radiation to a small rectal patch at the back of the prostate, this area may undergo a radiation reaction that can cause intermittent rectal bleeding. The bleeding may show up as a red spot on the toilet paper after a bowel movement, which can irritate rectal lining. Some minor rectal bleeding may occur in less than 5% of men, and only rarely requires medication. It usually clears up by itself in 12 to 24 months.

More serious rectal complications requiring surgical repair occur in less than 1% of all patients. Some men develop an ulceration of the rectum that can take a year or two to heal. In these cases, stool softeners, steroid enemas or anti-inflammatory drugs may be utilized. Reconstructive surgery (colostomy) is rarely necessary.

Sexual Symptoms and Complications

The prostate gland functions to provide fluid to help transport sperm. As such, radiation can affect sexual function, either temporarily, or in some cases, permanently. Sexual problems can include impotence (erectile dysfunction), pain during ejaculation, and blood in the semen.

About thirty percent of patients experience some brief discomfort or a burning sensation during ejaculation. These symptoms may persist 3 to 6 months after treatment. Over time, many men notice that they have less fluid with ejaculation, and the color of the ejaculate fluid may change, becoming more clear. Patients who may want to have children later are advised to bank their sperm before undergoing implantation.

Implantation can cause sexual impotence, which is defined as an inability to achieve or sustain an erection sufficient for intercourse (while desire for sex remains unchanged). While impotence is less likely to occur with seeding than with either surgery or external radiation, it can develop over time. Less than 5 percent of men become impotent within one year of treatment. At 5 years, approximately 25 percent of men become impotent, reflecting both the effect of radiation and the natural effects of aging. When it occurs, radiation-induced impotence apparently results from damage to the nerves and blood vessels responsible for erections.

In contrast, as many as 50 to 75 percent of surgical patients are permanently impotent after treatment, even with the nerve-sparing operation developed by Dr. Patrick Walsh of Johns Hopkins Hospital. This surgical technique attempts to preserve the nerve bundles that run along the back of the prostate gland and control erection. For men who are concerned about preserving potency, it should be underscored that a significantly larger percentage of patients retain potency with seed implantation compared to patients who are treated surgically, or with conventional external radiation.

Loss of potency after treatment is most often due to the treatment itself rather than psychological factors. In some cases, however, sexual potency may be impaired by psychological stress, anxiety, or depression. In these cases, a therapist should be consulted. A number of effective remedies are available for those patients who become impotent after any form of treatment. Remedies include oral drugs, injections, penile implants, and vacuum devices.

HOW ARE PATIENTS MONITORED AFTER SEEDING?

Patients are monitored with the PSA test and occasionally by biopsy. After implantation, a patient's PSA usually falls to low levels, and stays there over time if the treatment has been successful. The PSA may be checked every 3 to 4 months during the first year after treatment, and every 6 months thereafter. If the PSA rises, there is some risk of recurrence, and further testing, including a biopsy, may be called for. Some physicians use the biopsy as a matter of course for follow-up after 18-24 months, when the implant is no longer active.

The PSA valuation criteria used to assess cure with radiation therapy, including seed implants, are somewhat different from those which are used to evaluate surgical results. With surgery, since the prostate has been removed, the PSA is expected to drop to zero and stay there if a cure has been achieved. With radiation, since the prostate gland is still present, some PSA is expected, usually less than 1.0. That is the rigorous standard for cure now accepted by most physicians.

TEMPORARY IMPLANTS

Most of the considerations involved with permanent implants apply to temporary implants as well. A patient who is a candidate for permanent seeding would also be a candidate for the temporary implantation procedure. The temporary seeding procedure is generally combined with a course of low dose external radiation.

As with permanent seeding, the temporary procedure begins with comprehensive planning, often utilizing MRI images of the prostate. The patient has a choice of local or general anesthesia. Once the anesthesia takes effect, a catheter is inserted through the penis, and hollow tubes are inserted through the skin of the perineum. A plastic template is sewn into place and used to guide the tubes, through which the iridium isotope is inserted. Using ultrasound and X-rays, the physician calculates exactly how long the radioactive source is to be left in place. This calculation is known as "dwell time." Several exposure sessions may be necessary.

Typically, a patient will remain in the hospital from 2 to 5 days, during which the patient must remain in bed as motionless as possible to avoid moving the tubes. The advantage of the procedure is that it allows the physician to maximize the dose and duration of the exposure, while minimizing the temporary side effects associated with permanent implants.

Because temporary implants are used less frequently, few studies have yet been published, though it stands to reason that results would be comparable to those obtained with permanent implants. However, complication rates may be higher because of the more penetrating radiation involved with temporary implants.

COMMON QUESTIONS AND ANSWERS ABOUT SEEDING

1. I have been advised by my urologist to have a radical prostatectomy to treat my early stage, localized prostate cancer -- am I also a candidate for seeding?

If you are a candidate for radical surgery, you are most likely also a candidate for seeding.

2. What tests are conducted before seeding?

Prior to seeding, either an MRI or CT scan (or both) may be used to create an image of the prostate that the physician can use to plan the precise number and placement of the seeds. These tests are continually being refined, as new and more sophisticated equipment is brought into use, enabling physicians to more accurately visualize the tumor.

3. How long the does the procedure take, and how long will I be in the hospital?

The procedure usually takes only an hour, and the patient can be released from the hospital the same day. Some physician and hospital protocols may call for an overnight stay. After release, the patients can usually return to work and resume normal activities, although most doctors recommend that patients not engage in any excessive strenuous activities, such as heavy lifting, for a few days after the procedure.

4. Who will be in the operating room?

The physician (a urologist and/or radiation oncologist) and the nursing staff necessary to perform the procedure.

5. Will I be given a catheter? Why?

During the procedure, a catheter is inserted through the penis and into the bladder for drainage. The catheter helps to prevent urine retention, and is usually removed a short time after the procedure is complete.

6. How many seeds will I get?

Depending on the radiation dose required by your individual case, and by the type of isotope used, you might receive anywhere from 50 to 150 seeds.

7. Will prior health problems (heart, cancer, etc.) prevent me from qualifying for treatment?

In many cases, prior health problems will not prevent a patient from undergoing the seed implant procedure, but you may be asked to have additional tests, such as a cardiac stress test. You should always inform your physician about prior medical conditions.

8. What happens if I have an enlarged prostate?

If the prostate gland is larger than 60 cubic centimeters, your doctor may prescribe hormonal therapy for several months to shrink the prostate. If the gland cannot be reduced enough in size to qualify for seeding, your doctor may suggest another curative therapy, such as conformal radiation or prostatectomy.

9. What can be done to prepare for the seeding procedure?

The procedure may be better tolerated by men who have a healthy diet and exercise regime. Walking and Kegel exercises (sometimes described as trying to hold a dollar bill between the cheeks of the buttocks) may be beneficial.

10. What types of seeds are used most commonly, and what are the differences?

For permananent seed implants, the most commonly used isotopes are palladium (Pd-103) and iodine (I-125). Palladium has a shorter half-life than iodine, and therefore, delivers its radiation dose over a shorter period of time. Palladium may be more effective as a cure against larger, faster-growing tumors. Temporary side effects such as urinary distress and rectal irritation may not last as long with palladium because of its shorter half-life.

11. With seeding, will I need to give or receive blood?

Because the procedure is non-invasive, patients do not need to give or receive blood.

12. Is there an incision?

No. The seeding procedure involves only the insertion of needles, which implant the seeds in the prostate.

13. What objections to seeding are raised by doctors?

Many surgeons raise objections that seeding is still relatively new, and that the results are still too short-term. The fact is that seeding has been around for many years, and the improved results over the past decade have been dramatic. While it is true that these results are still considered short-term at 5 years, it should be noted that results with seeding are comparable or superior to results with surgery or external radiation, when compared at similar times.

14. Will I need a home care nurse after seeding?

No. The initial recovery usually only takes a day or two. Most patients resume work and other normal activities within that time.

15. How many patients have trouble with urination after the procedure, and what can be done about it?

Most patients experience some temporary urinary problems that may last from a few months to as long as a year, depending on the isotope used, the size of the prostate, the location of the tumor, the number of seeds, and so forth. These symptoms are usually most severe from 4 to 6 weeks after the procedure. A number of medications, such as Hytrin, Pyridium, Urised, Cardura and Levbid, are used to relieve urinary discomfort and frequency. Ibuprofen is also commonly prescribed for pain. A half teaspoon of baking soda added to an 8 ounce glass of cranberry juice may also be helpful. At least two glasses a day are recommended for the period immediately following the procedure.

16. How long will it be before my PSA goes down after the procedure?

The implantation causes trauma and swelling of the gland that may cause the PSA to rise or remain at an elevated level immediately after the seeding procedure. For this reason, most doctors wait 3 months before beginning to monitor the PSA. From that point, a downward trend should be established. The standard for cure is a PSA of 1.0 or less. The time for the PSA to drop to its lowest level varies widely from 1-2 years.

17. Does the same doctor who performed the procedure also have to monitor me afterwards?

No. Monitoring can be done by a local urologist or oncologist.

18. Can spinal anesthesia cause headaches or problems with the lower limbs?

Not usually. Such problems have been eliminated for the most part with the use of small needles and more precise delivery of the anesthetic. Most patients who undergo local or spinal anesthesia remain unaware of the insertion of various needles and probes during the procedure, and do not experience much discomfort.

19. Can radioactive seeds impair fertility?

Yes. Patients who wish to father children are advised to bank sperm prior to undergoing the procedure.

20. What temporary symptoms or side effects can I expect the first week, the first month, the first 6 months, the first year?

During the first week, you may experience some soreness in the perineal area where the needles were inserted. After the first week or so, there may be temporary urinary (burning, increased frequency, etc.), or rectal symptoms. Urinary symptoms usually peak at 4 to 6 weeks and gradually disappear over the next 3 to 12 months. Rectal irritation may begin within 2 to 3 weeks of the implant, and gradually disappears over 3 to 6 months. There also may be some temporary discomfort associated with ejaculation. For a full discussion of these temporary side effects, see above under "What Happens after the Procedure?"

21. What follow-up tests can I expect, and how frequently?

Patients are monitored with the PSA blood test and occasionally biopsy. PSA testing is done every 3 to 4 months during the first year after treatment, and every 6 months after that.

22. What happens if my PSA rises?

Your doctor will probably recommend further tests, such as a biopsy, to determine whether or not there is a recurrence of the cancer, and if so, how far it has spread. While recurrence is not good news, there are still a number of options available to treat a recurrent cancer after seeding.

23. What happens if I have a recurrence?

If cancer should recur after seeding, your treatment options can include surgery (prostatectomy), reseeding (if failure resulted from misplacement of the seeds), hormones, orchiectomy, and watchful waiting. For a full discussion of recurrence, readers are referred to the Survivor's Guide Booklet entitled, "Recurrence: What do I do Now?"

24. When will my sex life return?

Most patients can resume normal sexual relations within 1 to 2 months after seeding.

25. What medications are prescribed after the procedure?

Medications are typically prescribed to prevent any possibility of infection, and to treat any temporary urinary or rectal symptoms that may arise.

26. What happens to the seeds inside the body?

The seeds become intert and inactive over time, depending on the amount of time that it takes for the particular isotope used to give off its radiation dose (12 months with iodine versus 3 months with palladium). Seeds remaining in the body are harmless.

27. How will my semen change?

After seeding, the ejaculate fluid that carries the sperm may become more clear in color, and there may be less fluid.

28. What is the risk of permanent side effects with seeding?

Less than 1 percent of patients experience urinary incontinece or serious rectal damage. There may be a higher risk of urinary incontinence for men with a prior TURP. Approximately 20-25 percent of men will develop impotence within five years after treatment, depending on age and health. Men over 60 are somewhat more likely to experience problems with potency.

29. Will I feel the seeds?

No. You will not be aware of the seeds after they are implanted.

30. If I travel will I set off security devices?

No. The seeds are not large enough to be detected by security devices.

31. Do I need to tell my airline that I have recently been seeded?

No.

32. Will sitting be difficult?

Not usually. There may be soreness, and sitting may be uncomfortable for a week or so after the procedure. Ibuprofen often helps alleviate the problem.

33. What are "Rapid Strands?

A braided strand of suture material is sometimes used with iodine implants to prevent the seeds from migrating during and after the procedure. These are known as rapid strands, and special needles are used to insert them. They are not available with palladium or with temporary implants. It is not clear that the rapid strands offer any great advantage, as the migration of seeds is rarely problematic.

34. What treatments are used in conjunction with seeding?

Hormonal therapy may be used for 2 to 3 months prior to seeding to debulk the tumor. Low dose external radiation may be used with seeding (either before or after) for high risk patients. When the dose and delivery of the radiation is tailored to the patient using hi-tech methods, it is known as conformal radiation therapy.

35. If the doctor wants to include a course of external radiation, does that mean I have a more serious case?

Seeding is combined with external radiation when there is a higher risk that the cancer has spread beyond the prostate capsule. Such a risk is indicated by a PSA of 10 or higher, or a combined Gleason score of 7 or higher, or an elevated PAP, or a clinical stage of T2B or higher. Early results with combining seed implants with external (conformal) radiation appear promising, and may prove to be more effective than either seeding alone or external radiation alone for high risk patients.

36. How much time is needed between external radiation and seeds?

When combining external radiation and seeding, most doctors start the seed implant 2 to 6 weeks after completion of the course of external radiation. There are a few physicians who do the reverse, first implanting the seeds and then starting the course external radiation.

37. Regarding conformal radiation, how many treatments of what dosage are required over what period of time?

Radiation is given in small daily doses five days a week, usually over a period of 7 to 8 weeks. Conventional external radiation usually involves a dose of approximately 70 Gray. With conformal radiation, the dose is more highly focused and delivered more accurately and safely; and therefore, a dose of 75 Gray or higher may be used.

38. Will my doctor provide me with names of other patients he has treated?

Most doctors will be willing to refer you to other patients who have undergone the procedure. It is wise to talk to others who have gone the route so you know exactly what to expect.

39. How should I choose a doctor to perform the seed implant procedure? Are some doctors better than others in the same way that some surgeons are more skilled than others.

There are now several hundred doctors using seeds at various medical centers around the country. You should try to find an experienced physician with whom you communicate well. Ask your doctor how many procedures he has performed, where he was trained for the procedure, and what his success rate is. Because of the technical expertise required, results among doctors using seeds may vary in the same way that results among surgeons and other specialists may vary.

40. How do I find a qualified doctor who is experienced in seeding?

A list of doctors using palladium is available from the Theragenics Corporation by calling 1-800-458-4372. A list of doctors using iodine is available from the Medi-Physics Corporation by calling 1-708-593-6300.

CONCLUSION

As of August 1996, the results of clinical studies on seeding (alone and combined with external radiation) have reached 7 years, and appear comparable or superior to results with radical surgery, but with significantly less morbidity. As such, more and more men are choosing seeding, and the implant procedure is now becoming available at an ever increasing number of hospitals and medical centers throughout the country.

If you are a patient confronted with the choice of treatment, please contact the Prostate Cancer Resource Network with your questions and concerns. Members of the Network will be happy to direct you to other patients who have been through the procedure and can help you evaluate your options and prepare for therapy.

If you are a patient who has undergone the seed implant procedure, you can help others by becoming an "Encourager" - counseling other patients who are embarking on the same path through our Outreach Program.

In the years ahead, we expect seeding to become the gold standard for the treatment of early stage prostate cancer, and you - fellow patients - can help by becoming involved and offering your support through the foundation.

**To be a cancer survivor,
you must first be a cancer fighter!**

GLOSSARY

Anesthetic. A drug that produces general or local loss of physical sensations, particularly pain. A "spinal" is the injection of a local anesthetic into the area surrounding the spinal cord.

Biopsy. A procedure involving the removal of tissue from the body of the patient. Removed tissue is typically examined microscopically by a pathologist in order to make a precise diagnosis of the patient's condition.

Brachytherapy (seed implantation). A form of radiation therapy in which radioactive seeds are implanted into the prostate to deliver radiation directly to the tumor.

Cancer. A cellular malignancy typically forming tumors. Unlike benign tumors, these tend to invade surrounding tissues and spread to distant sites of the body.

Chemotherapy. The treatment of cancer using chemicals that deter the growth of cancer cells.

Combination Therapy. A form of hormonal therapy that surgically or chemically blocks the production of testosterone by the testes, and involves the additional use of an antiandrogen to block the receptor sites from utilizing testosterone produced by the adrenal glands.

Conformal. A treatment conforming precisely to the size and shape of the prostate, with the use of computerized planning and state-of-the-art imaging techniques.

Diagnosis. Evlauation of a patient's symptoms and/or test results, with the intent of identifying and verifying the existence of any underlying disease or abnormal condition.

Digital Rectal Examination (DRE). A procedure in which the physician inserts a gloved, lubricated finger into the rectum to examine the prostate gland for signs of cancer.

Gleason Score. A widely used method for classifying the cellular differentiation of cancerous tissue. The less the cancerous cells appear like normal cells, the more malignant the cancer. Two grades of 1-5, identifying the two most common degrees of differentiation present in the examined tissue sample, are added together to produce the Gleason score.

Hormonal Therapy. Cancer treatment involving the blockage of hormone production by surgical or chemical means. Because prostate cancer is usually dependent on male hormones to grow, hormonal therapy can be an effective means of alleviating symptoms and retarding the development of the disease.

Impotence. The loss of ability to produce and/or sustain an erection (while desire for sex remains unchanged).

Incontenence. A loss of urinary control. There are various kinds and degrees of incontinence. *Overflow incontinence* is a condition in which the bladder retains urine after voiding. As a consequence, the bladder remains full most of the time, resulting in involuntary seepage of urine from the bladder. *Stress incontinence* is the involuntary discharge of urine when there is increased pressure upon the bladder, as in coughing or straining to lift heavy objects. *Total incontinence* is the failure of ability to voluntarily exercise control over the sphincters of the bladder neck and urethra, resulting in total loss of retentive ability.

Inflammation. Redness or swelling caused by injury or infection.

Lymph Node. A small bean-shaped mass of tissue along the vessels of the lymphatic system. The lymph nodes filter out bacteria and other toxins, as well as cancer cells.

Metastasis. The spread of cancer, by way of the blood stream or lymphatic system, beyond the boundaries of the organ or structure where the cancer originated. *Metastases* is the plural.

Morbidity. Unhealthy consequences and complications resulting from treatment.

Perineum. The area of the body between the anus and scrotum. A perineal procedure uses this area as the point of entry into the body.

Prognosis. The forecast of the course of a disease, and future prospects of the patient.

Progression. A change in the status of the cancer indicating the condition has progressed and worsened.

Prostate Specific Antigen (PSA). A blood test that measures a substance manufactured solely by prostate gland cells. An elevated reading indicates an abnormal condition of the prostate gland, either benign or malignant. It is presently the most sensitive tumor marker for the identification and monitoring of prostate cancer.

Prostatic Acid Phosphatase (PAP). An enzyme produced by the prostate that is elevated in many patients when prostate cancer has spread beyond the prostate.

Favor - Adamson - Nurse for
     Conrad
11:30

East Side of Hospital   Parking Rear
    Room   or East
Emergency Side
me in Center door
    curtain down hall says
        green sign — Surgical
    Maris from center   Services

Dress Casually.   Bring
Case for glasses.   Suitcase
                            in later.

Clear liquid
Black Coffee | No Milk
Tea | No orange juice
Water

papers known Pre op - physical

              '924 5188
              for question

Christmas Truck Plans

T-Tim 7:00 - will call
    tomorrow

Radiation Therapy. Use of high energy rays to kill cancer cells.

Radical Prostatectomy. An operation to remove the entire prostate gland and seminal vesicles.

Recurrence. Return of the cancer following remission or treatment intended as curative. Local recurrence indicates a return of the cancer at the site of origin. Distant recurrence indicates the appearance of one or more metatases of the disease.

Staging. The testing process by which the extent and severity of a known cancer is evaluated according to an established system of classification. It is used to help determine appropriate therapy.

Transurethral Resection of the Prostate (TURP). A surgical procedure to remove tissue obstructing the urethra. The technique involves the insertion of an instrument called a resectoscope into the penile urethra, and is intended to relieve obstruction of urine flow due to enlargement of the prostate.

Tumor. An excessive growth of cells caused by uncontrolled and disorderly cell replacement.

Urethra. The tube that carries urine from the bladder and semen from the prostate out of the body through the penis.

What Every Man Should Know About Seeding
Copyright 1996 by Prostate Cancer Resource Network

This Survivor's Guide Booklet is provided courtesy of the Prostate Cancer Resource Network. Suggested donation is $5.00/copy. For additional copies, please contact:

Prostate Cancer Resource Network
P.O. Box 966, New Port Richey, FL 34656
Telephone: (800) 580-6866
Fax: (813) 848-2494

For copies of Donald Kaltenbach's **PROSTATE CANCER: A SURVIVOR'S GUIDE**, please call toll free: (800) 580-6866.